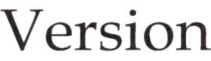

Be
Sex
Star II
A Greatly Expanded Version

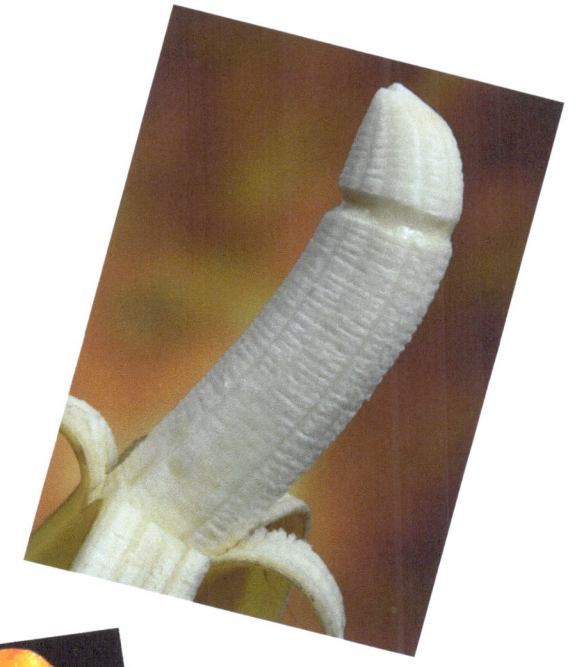

by Goshua Iem

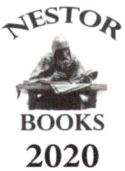

BOOKS
2020

Goshua Iem

Be sex star

The best original recipes for juices, smoothies and sweet-food for increased libido and sexual stamina
with juicy jokes for each recipe

by Goshua Iem

Table of Contents

Introduction..2
About Author...4
Juices and Smoothies 5
Bananas Smoothie "The Lasting Fruit"...................6
Avocado Smoothies "The Power Stream".............8
Special Pomegranate Juice "Big Red Head".........9
Maca Smoothie "The Harem of Montezuma"....10
Beetroot Smoothie "The Pulsating Blood".........11
Watermelon Smoothies "The Inner Flesh"......... 14
Celery Smoothie "The Horse Stalk"......................16
Why did Julius Caesar and Cleopatra have a great sex?.17
Pumpkin and Hemp Seeds Smoothie "Two pouches".....18
Berries Smoothie "Ripe strawberries"..................19
Berries Smoothie "My Blueberry Nights"...........21
Carrots Smoothie "The Red Rod".........................23
Chocolate Smoothie "Black Supersex" 25
Sweet-food...26
Blueberry Brioche Rolls with Almond 27
Berries Oats Pudding..28
Blueberry Coffee Cake...29
Date Cake...30
Have a good sex...33

Introduction

It's a second part of the book. It contains more recipes. It means that you'll have more sex and pleasure!

One of the greatest things in the world is sex. Moreover, without doubts, it is one of the greatest pleasures in our life. However, we live fast and hard. This affects the quality of sex. We have fewer pleasures, less relaxation, and love.

For better satisfying our partners, we can take expensive medications. On the other hand, for example, visit sex therapists. However, we can also use the gifts of nature.

These are not silly recipes from the Internet. Goshua Iem gives only thorough tested smoothie recipes, which he has discussed with his friends in Asia and on various islands in the Pacific Ocean.

A distinctive feature of the book – jokes about every fruit and vegetable, from which we make a smoothie. We also warn people about threats. For example, many authors do not write that beet juice should settle in a glass for six hours or the fact that there is a dangerous toxin in the avocado's bones and peel.

With my diet, you will become more confident and stronger. You will be able to get rid of feelings of guilt and dissatisfaction. In addition, you will be very surprised to find out that juice diet played such a huge role in the bedroom.

Goshua Iem

About author

The author is the famous yogi and traveler Goshua Iem. He also has a black belt in karate Shotokan. He traveled to many eastern countries, where he gathered secrets of how to live young, joyful and happy.

This is how his collection was created. A part of it Goshua will share with his readers.

Goshua understands that in the modern world a person is in need of proper nutrition for excellent sexual stamina.

Therefore, he shares a variety of recipes.

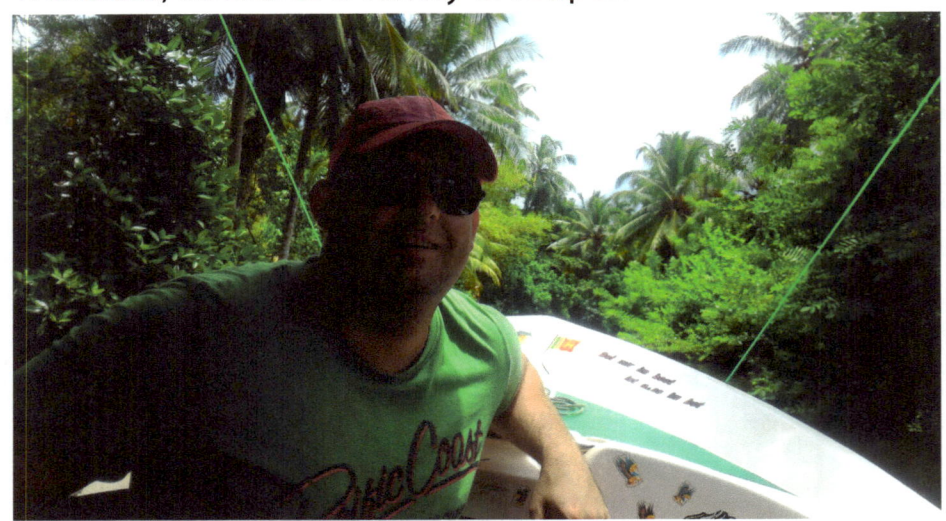

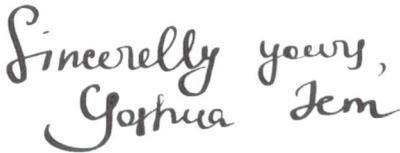

Juices and Smoothies

Young people often don't have enough energy, vitamins and the power of nature. In the same time, many persons in the age of 40+ have decreased hormonal production. The processes of blood oxidation influence the level of sexual activity. Besides, the juices can stable it.

Moreover, you can say that you drink juices just for the sake of a healthy diet. No need to secretly take pills or visit a doctor. However, your partner will soon appreciate your achievements in sex.

In this book, we present recipes for juices and smoothies that will enhance your libido. The juice mixes consist of the main ingredient and auxiliary components. The effect will be great.

One of the objectives of this book is to make many sexual contacts successful.

We do not promise that one glass of juice prepared according to our recipe will make you Apollos or Venus. However, using our juices for at least few weeks will make your sex life better.

Let's get started!

Goshua Iem

Bananas Smoothie "The Lasting Fruit"

A banana is a phallic symbol. Therefore, it can't be not useful for quality sex. First, bananas are aphrodisiacs. Secondly, it is a powerful source of energy. Thirdly, it provides sexual stamina. Bananas also increase serotonin level it makes you more joyful and resourceful. Believe me our Smoothie is very tasty. You can treat your soul mate.

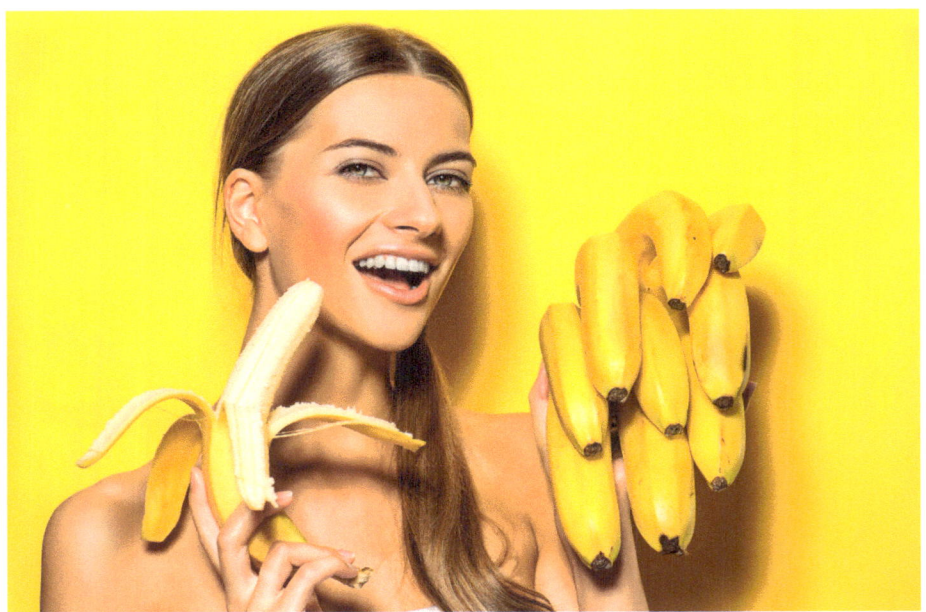

Joke:
- How much does this banana cost? - 5 francs, madam - How do you know that I am madam, not mademoiselle? - You are holding this banana in this way...

Our cocktail contains life important elements. For example, chemical dopamine, zinc, magnesium and vitamin B6, all of which have an effect on improving your mood. And your phallus will be in the form of a banana.

This fruit is naturally free of fat, cholesterol, and sodium. One serving of banana is considered to be about 126 grams. So, it contains:

Ingredients:

- 150 ml cup reduced fat milk
- 1 banana
- 2 tablespoons yoghurt
- ½ teaspoon cinnamon
- 4 ice cubes
- 1 tablespoon honey
- 1 tablespoon chia seeds
- few raw cashews
- juiced lemon
- 100 ml of clean water

Directions:

- Add the juiced lemon
- Place all ingredients in blender and process until smooth
- Add water
- Pour into glass and serve immediately.

Goshua Iem

Avocado Smoothies "The Power Stream"

Avocado is a real super battery from an intergalactic spacecraft. As we know, energy is needed in the bedroom. Avocado possesses such qualities due to its high content of folic acids. Healthy fats, Vitamin B and potassium, which are also found in avocados, are involved in the production of male hormones. That increases libido too.

Ingredients:

- 2 large balls of avocado (don't forget to remove the seeds and peel)
- ¼ pineapple
- 70 ml almond milk
- 15 grams of ginger
- 1 pear
- 1 red apple
- 100 ml clean water

Directions:

- Place the avocado, the pineapple, the apple and the pear in blender and process until smooth
- Add the ginger and the almond milk
- Add water
- Mix one more time
- Pour into glass and drink.

But be careful, the leaves, the skin of the fruit and the avocado bone contain the fungicidal toxin - persin. This toxin is dangerous for both animals and humans. Therefore, you have to peel the avocado.

Joke:
Two friends are talking.
A: How to know that avocado is ripe?
B: For men, this is not a problem! We all know how elastic our penis is during an erection, so if an avocado has the same elasticity, then it is ripe.
A: Does it mean, you are in the store choosing avocados with one hand on the shelf, and the other - in the pants?.. (putting the hand in the pants) Ha! How do I split such a hard avocado?

Special Pomegranate Juice "Big Red Head"

Known thing to enhance libido. A daily glass of pomegranate juice as study shows boosts our sexual desire. It provides a real "Viagra effect".

Pomegranate juice contains antioxidants that will make your sexual stamina better. This juice also has a good effect on the heart and blood vessels. Which, as we know, play a significant role during sex.

Goshua Iem
_____

Scientists recently conducted research at Queen Margaret University (Edinburgh). They found that pomegranate juice increases testosterone levels.

Moreover, the scientist in in another study have identified, that pomegranate juice may help stop the growth of prostate cancer cells.

Ingredients:

- 300 grams of seeded pomegranates
- 20 grams of fresh ginger
- ½ of lemon
- 1 tablespoon honey
- 150 ml of water

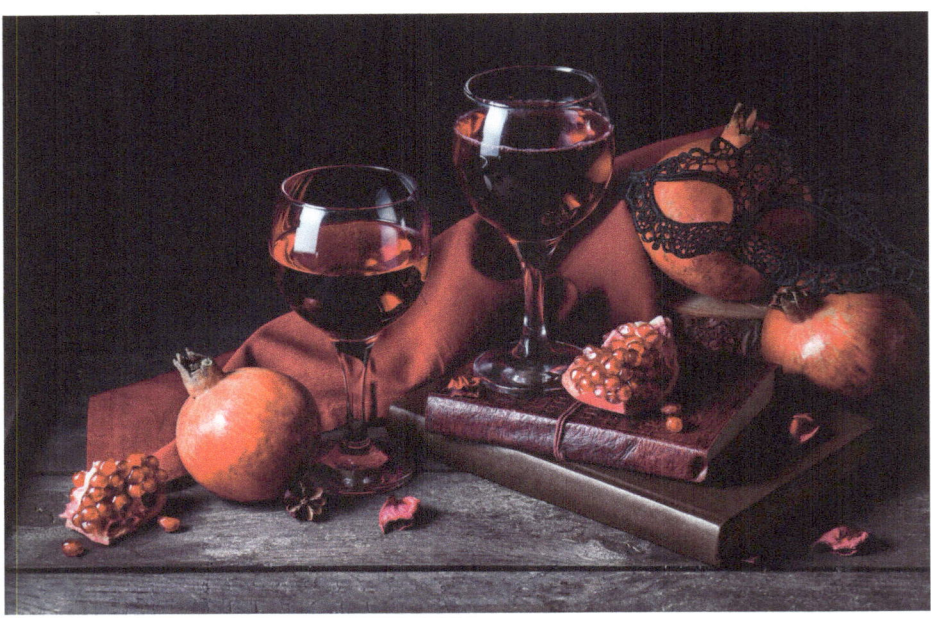

Directions:

- Put the seeded pomegranates in a blender
- Add chopped ginger
- Add the juiced lemon
- Add a cup of water
- Blend all the ingredients
- I recommend adding the ice to the glass

Joke:
I like juice - it is an endless source of vitamins and trace elements in my alcohol.

Maca Smoothie
"The Harem of Montezuma"

This plant grows in the Andes. A strong aphrodisiac improves the sexual functions of men and women. It is difficult to get it fresh, but the food stores sell powdered maca.

Peruvian Indians knew about the healing possibilities of maca and used it as food. The grandees used the powder maca before enjoying sex with their concubines in harems.

Goshua Iem

Ingredients:

- 1 apple
- 1 teaspoon of maca
- 1/2 cup skim milk
- 1 tablespoon sport protein powder
- 1/2 peeled banana
- 10 grams ginger.

Direction:

- Place all the ingredients into blender
- Add the grated ginger, milk and protein
- Blend it all together until smooth
- Add maca
- Drink.

Joke:
Q: What does a frash maca have in common with good sex?
A: They're both very rare.

Beetroot Smoothie
"The Pulsating Blood"

It is known that beetroot juice has been used to increase the erectile functions for several millennia. Therefore, representatives of all classes: from emperors to workers drank it. Later, scientists found that it is useful, primarily because there is a lot of vitamin C, folate (B9) – one of the B-vitamins, magnesium, iron and potassium in beets.

The beets also contain other chemical components that perfectly affect the overall health and libido in particular. They break down to nitric oxide. This is a very interesting thing in the context of improving the quality of sex. This substance affects the body of a man like Viagra. It, basically, pumps blood into the penis. It becomes hard and inflexible.

Understandably, there are no by-effects from beet juice. But there is one caveat. The juice has to stand a long time. For example, you did your magic juice in evening, so you may drink it in the morning. Yes, bro, just before invigorating morning sex.

Joke:
- Are you stealing my beets?
- Of course not. I pull it up for the beets grow faster.

Ingredients:
- 1 beetroot
- 1 green apple
- 2 Medium sized celery stalks
- 15 grams of fresh ginger
- ½ of lemon
- 200 ml of clean water

Directions:
- Peel all the vegetables
- Cut them into small pieces
- Throw it all into a blender or juicer
- Add water to the mixture, mix abd drink

Goshua Iem

Watermelon Smoothies
"The Inner Flesh"

Watermelon is not only tasty and refreshing. It contains Citrulline, which, on the one hand, relaxes, and on the other – dilates blood vessels. Citrulline converts to arginine, the amino acid, which that has such an effect.

This fruit improves blood flow to erectile tissue, of which the penis and the clitoris are made. So drink our smoothies together.

But for ladies there is a recommendation. If woman wants to get pregnant, she shouldn't drink a lot of watermelon smoothie.

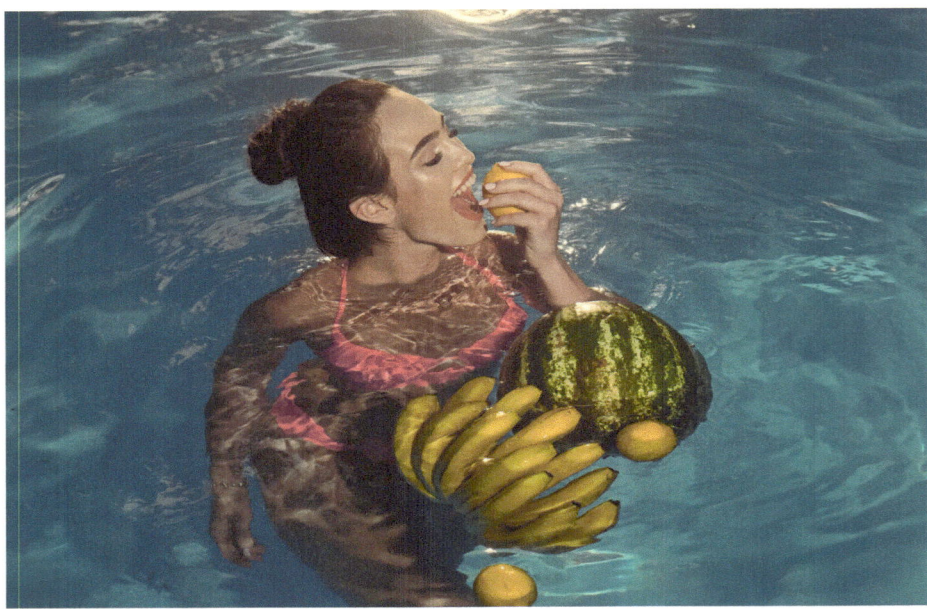

Ingredients:

- 250 gram of watermelon with the seeds
- 1 piece of apple
- 15 grams of ginger
- 70 ml of almond milk
- 50 ml of yoghurt without sugar
- 1 tablespoon of honey.

Directions:

- Place the watermelon and the apple into blender
- Add the grated ginger, milk and yoghurt
- Blend it all together until smooth
- Drink.

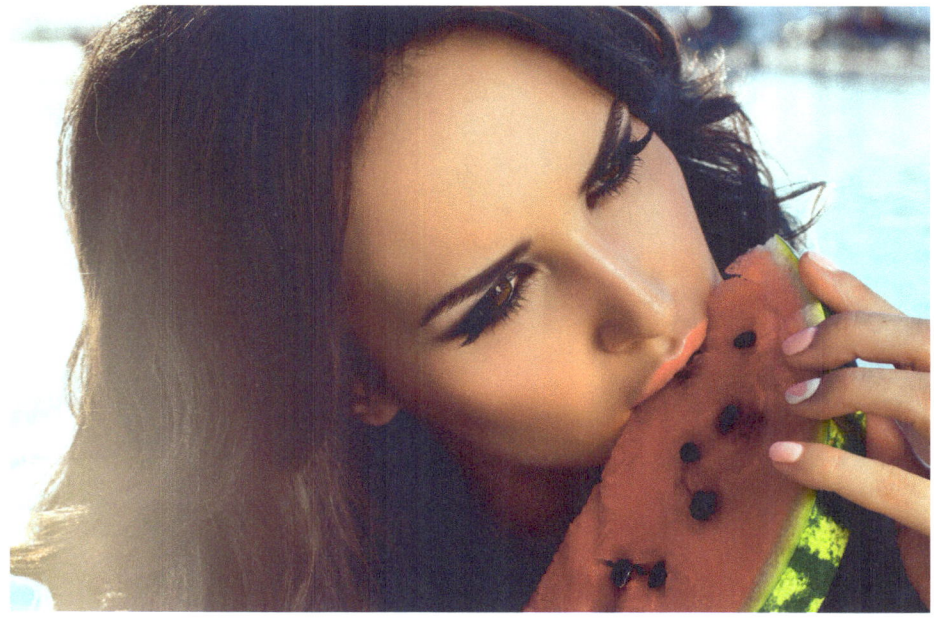

Joke:
- *How are you?*
- *Like a watermelon ...*
- *???*
- *The belly grows, and the tip dries out!*

Celery Smoothie "The Horse Stalk"

Celery contains sodium, which makes the body younger. It contains many minerals and vitamin C, which – in addition to increase of sexual stimulation in men – helps maintain skin elasticity.

Ingredients:

- 3 stalk of celery
- 1 apple
- 1 cup spinach
- 1/2 thumb tip ginger root
- 1/2 Avocado
- 100 ml of clean water
- 1 tablespoon honey

Directions:

- Peel the lemon, lime, and ginger
- Process all ingredients in a juicer
- Shake or stir
- Serve.

Joke:
Dialogue in the restaurant:
- What do you advice?
- I would advise you celery and carrots.
- That is you who are fat!

Why did Julius Caesar and Cleopatra have a great sex?

I want to say you few words about the **saffron**. Saffron is a spice that has a very good effect on libido and sexual stamina. And the ancient people knew it. We know Julius Caesar added saffron to rice and meat. He also put some saffron in the tea.

Everyone knows that Cleopatra bathed in goat milk. She did it for skin care. But not everyone knows that before meeting with her lovers, she took a bath of saffron decoction.

The ancient Romans even had a tradition to sprinkle the bed of newlywed's with saffron. They knew that after it, the man would have an excellent erection, and the woman would get multiple orgasms.

Saffron is a powerful aphrodisiac that affects not only men, but also women. Moreover, saffron is a useful antioxidant. It relaxes your mind, helps with insomnia and woman's PMS. Therefore, I recommend adding saffron to your smoothies.

Goshua Iem

Pumpkin and Hemp Seeds Smoothie "Two pouches"

Seeds usually contain various useful elements in a concentrated manner. We need those that will increase sexual stamina and make us the sex star. I propose a smoothie recipe based on two types of seeds: pumpkin and hemp.

Pumpkin Seeds are high in zinc. It has a positive effect on hormones, including prevention of testosterone deficiency in men.

In addition, it improves sperm production and quality. Pumpkin seeds contain the minerals and vitamins that are most needed for quality sex like vitamins: B, E, C, D, K; minerals: potassium, phosphorous, and calcium.

In hemp seeds, we find a large amount of Omega-3 fatty acids and proteins. It also has L-arginine. All this together has a very positive effect on the production of male hormones (like testosterone).

Joke:
At midnight, Cinderella turned into a pumpkin. Nevertheless, the prince was already unstoppable.

Ingredients:

- 100 ml coconut milk
- 1 teaspoon powdered
- 1 banana
- ½ of apple
- 1 tablespoon pumpkin seeds
- 1 tablespoon hemp seeds
- 2 tablespoons cashew butter or 50 gram raw cashews
- 10 gram fresh ginger
- ½ teaspoon of cinnamon
- 1 tablespoon honey.

Direction:

- Add all ingredients into your blender
- Blend until smooth
- Drink the nostrum.

Berries Smoothie "Ripe strawberries"

It's no wonder that berries always were a delicacy. Little fruit like strawberry, raspberry, and currant (now widely produced in California) contains Vitamin C and E, anti-oxidants, ellagic acid (has some ability to slow the growth of cancer cells and to promote proper blood flow, including in genitals), beta carotene, zinc, iron, potassium, pro biotics and natural sugars.
Almost all of these components improve the libido in one or another way.

Goshua Iem

Ingredients:

- A handful of fresh strawberries
- A handful of fresh raspberries and currants
- 100 gram pineapple
- 1 tablespoon of honey
- 70 ml of fatty yogurt

Direction:

- Pour all inside your blender
- Just blend it and drink
- Have a strong sex.

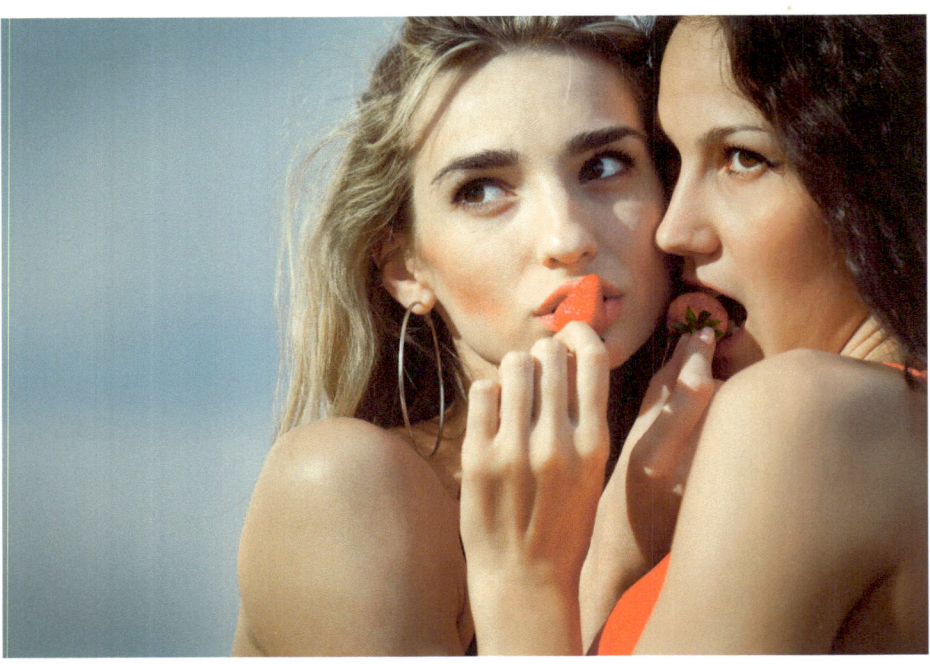

Joke:
Recently, classmates called me to the country, and for the first time in my life I worked in the garden. I had torn off strawberry runners all the day and I tanned much. Tell me, is it really necessary to do this naked, or else the strawberries will not grow?

Berries Smoothie "My Blueberry Nights"

In continuation of the berry theme. Blueberry is associated with health, sex and pleasure not without reason. This berry is full of free-radical scavenging antioxidants and phytonutrients, which promote your health. Blueberries contain calcium-D-glucarat and resveratrol (anti-aging and disease-fighting power).

All of these components counteract the excessive production of estrogen and provide a positive hormonal balance in your body.
In principle, blueberries, fresh or frozen, can be used to make smoothies. The lack of blueberries - if you eat a lot of it, there will be constipation.

In this smoothie we add coconut oil, which contains some saturated fats. These fats are involved in the production of the male hormone testosterone. As a bonus, it can also normalize weight.

Goshua Iem

Ingredients:

- ½ a cup of blueberries
- A handful of currants
- 20-30 gram sour cream
- 2 peeled walnuts
- 1 ½ tablespoon of coconut oil
- 70 ml low-fat yogurt
- 50 ml coconut milk
- 50 ml clean water

Direction:

- Place the blueberries, the currants, the pear in blender and process until smooth
- Add walnuts, coconut oil, the yogurt, the sour cream and the coconut milk in blender
- Add water
- Mix one more time
- Pour into glass and drink.

Joke:
Few know that if give Viagra to the snake, in skillful hands it is as dangerous as a knife.

Carrots Smoothie "The Red Rod"

Carrots have a great effect on the skin and boosts immune system. This is due to carotenoids which physiological role is that of antioxidants, preventing oxidative stress and enhancing the immune system.

In addition, there is lot of beta-carotene in carrots. Because of this, it improves the ability of sperm fluids to swim. Men who eat carrots have better sperm motility.

Everybody knows it. However, this one increases libido and improves your hard-on. If the ancient Romans used saffron to improve sex, the ancient Greeks knew the secret of carrots. However, they once thought carrots were the secret to great sex.

This is well-known for us libido enhancer, it is loaded with Vitamin A, which is also found in large quantities in carrots, it helps produce more male hormones. Because of that a man becomes more passionate and hardy.

Joke:
In a nunnery. The abbess says: - Today for lunch we'll have a carrot. - Waxing joy. - Do not rejoice, it will be rubbed.

Goshua Iem

Ingredients:

- 200 grams of diced carrots
- 1 apple
- ½ cup of diced pineapples
- 15 grams of ginger
- 1 tablespoon of honey
- 70 ml yogurt (I recommend the fat one)
- 100 ml of clean water.

Direction:

- Pour your diced carrots into your blender
- Add apples and pineapples
- Add water and grated gingers
- Blend your ingredients together until smooth.

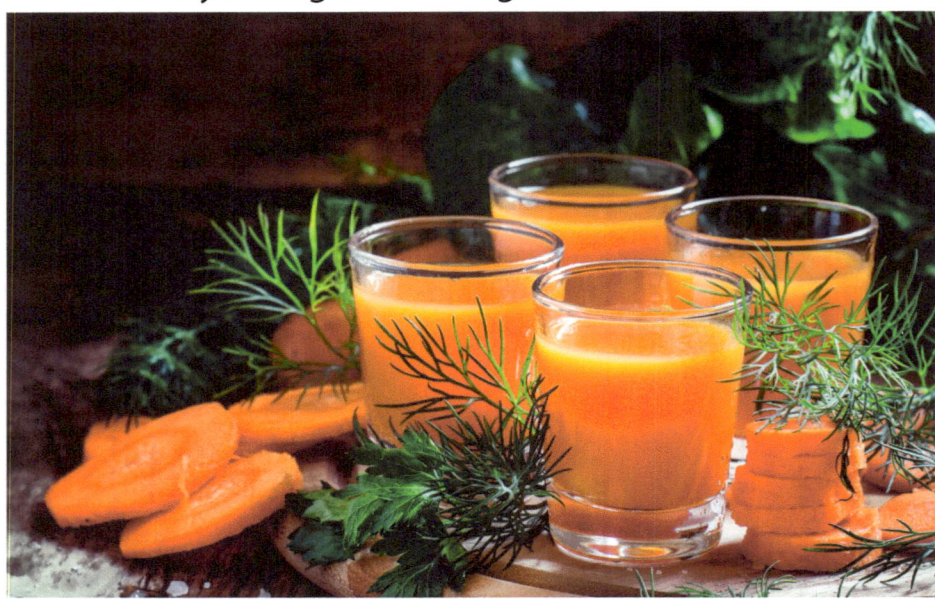

Chocolate Smoothie "Black Supersex"

I recommend to take only true black chocolate min 70%. You have to know, that dark chocolate increases the dopamine levels in your brain. It also has the neurotransmitter (for pleasure). Chocolate contains many antioxidants and the other components, which boost libido. Moreover, your life is better with chocolates.

Ingredients:

- 3 tablespoons dark chocolate (70% cocoa or more)
- ½ of banana
- ½ of peach
- 15-gram ginger
- A little bit mint
- 50 ml low-fat milk
- 50 ml clean water

Direction:

- Put ingredients in a blender until smooth
- Enjoy.

Joke:
Ben really wanted a chocolate bar, but he gave it to Julia, because he wanted Julia more.

Goshua Iem

Sweet-food

Blueberry Brioche Rolls with Almond

I do like those sexy berries. They help in the treatment and prevention of certain diseases. For example, when you catch a cold - vitamins contained in the blueberry, boost the immune system. Berry is good in the treatment of gallbladder and liver disease. And, of course, these berries are very good for the eyes. And it is perfect for sexual stamina.

Ingredients:

- 1/4 cup milk
- 1/4 cup white sugar
- 2 teaspoons dried yeast
- 2 cups plain bread flour
- 1/4 teaspoon salt
- 3 whisked eggs
- 1/2 cup butter, cut into 1/2 inche pieces
- 1/2 cup brown sugar
- 1/3 cup frozen or fresh blueberries
- 1 egg white
- 1 tablespoon white sugar
- 1/8 cup flaked almonds

Direction:

1. First we make the dough. Like real chefs, we do it ourselves. Mix and whisk the milk, white sugar and yeast in a tumbler. Place the flour and salt in a large bowl. Make a well in the center of flour and salt mixture slide. Add the yeast mixture and egg. Stir until a soft dough

forms. Turn onto a lightly floured surface and knead for 5 minutes. Do it well until smooth.
2. Add 2 pieces of butter to the dough and knead again. Knead in remaining butter, 2 pieces at a time, until dough is smooth and elastic. Place the dough in a large bowl. Cover with plastic wrap or clean light fabric. Set aside in a warm draught-free place to prove for 1 hour or until dough increase in size.
3. Punch down the dough. Roll out on a lightly floured surface to a 20 x 15 inches rectangle. Sprinkle with brown sugar and blueberries. Starting from the long end, roll up to enclose the filling. You have to trim the ends with a sharp knife. Cut into 10 even pieces. Place, cut-side up and just touching, in a flower shape on a large baking tray. Cover and set aside in a warm, draught-free place until rolls rise a little. It will take about 30 minutes.
4. Preheat oven to 360 degrees F (180 degrees C). Combine the egg white, almonds and white sugar in a bowl. Drizzle over the rolls. Bake, covering with foil, for 25-30 minutes or until the rolls are golden brown.
5. Bon appetite!

Joke:

Fox News is asked:
- Are there enough masks to protect against coronavirus?
- Not enough! A condom is also needed.

Berries Oats Pudding

Easy and fast breakfast, easy to cook and hard to sex. That's not sugary.
Regular consumption of these berries improves skin color, strengthens the immune system, stimulates the muscles of the intestines and improves digestion. Also, raspberries are used to treat viral diseases.

Ingredients:

- 4 cups rolled oats
- 1/2 cup coconut flakes
- 1/2 teaspoon ground cinnamon
- 1/2 teaspoon vanilla powder
- 1 1/2 teaspoons baking powder
- 3 eggs
- 1 1/2 cups milk
- 1 cup very finely grated apple
- 1/2 cup honey
- 1/2 cup frozen or fresh raspberries
- 1/2 cup frozen or fresh blueberries
- 1 tablespoon sunflower seed
- 1/4 cup chopped almond kernels
- 1 cup low-fat coconut yoghurt, to serve

Direction:
1. Preheat oven to 360 degrees F (180 degrees C). Grease 1.5 inches deep, 8 inches x 10 inches enamel baking

dish.
2. Place oats, coconut, ground cinnamon and vanilla powder mixture with baking powder in a bowl. Stir to combine.
3. Place eggs, milk, apple purée (very finely grated apple or from store) and honey in a medium bowl. Whisk to combine.
4. Add egg mixture to oat mixture. Stir to combine. Pour mixture into prepared baking dish. Sprinkle with berries, sunflower seed and almonds. Cook for 25 to 30 minutes or until golden and just set. Wait a few minutes. Drizzle your pudding with honey. You may serve it with yoghurt; I prefer to do like this.

Joke:
- What do you prefer - tea with raspberries or sex with a man?
- I don't care, if I sweat anyway.

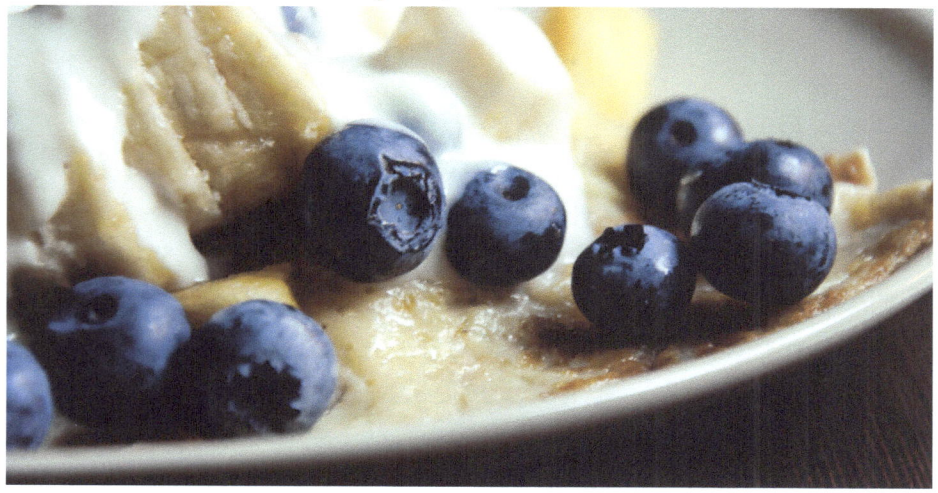

Goshua Iem

Blueberry Coffee Cake

The perfect and delicious moist cake with healthy blueberry. If you want, it is easy to throw together in the food processor. There are the milk, the blueberries and the nutmeg in a list of happy food.

Ingredients:
- 4 tablespoons butter
- 2 cups fresh blueberries (as a last resort take frozen)
- 2 cups flour
- 2 1/2 teaspoons baking powder
- 1/2 teaspoon salt
- 3/4 cup milk
- 2/3 cup sugar
- 2 eggs
- 2 tablespoons sugar (it is better to take brown)
- 1/4 teaspoon nutmeg

Direction:
1. Place flour, baking powder, salt and sugar into a food processor to sift and lighten.
2. Add in this mixture the softened butter and pulse again.
3. Then add milk and eggs. Pulse again.
4. Dust blueberries with flour. Mix in with your hands 2 cups of blueberries. Add also the nutmeg.
5. Bake in a 9-inch pan at 350 degrees F (180 degrees C) for 30 to 40 minute.
6. Let cool and be happy. Or be cool and let to be happy yourself.

Date Cake

A simple cake with few ingredients. I like this recipe. The dates contain a lot of magnesium, which our bodies will use for producing a mass of serotonin.
This is also not too sweet.

Ingredients:
- 3/4 cup butter
- 1 cup milk
- 1/2 cup brown sugar
- 1 cup chopped dates
- 1/2 teaspoon nutmeg
- 1/2 teaspoon bicarbonate of soda
- 1/2 teaspoon cinnamon
- 2 lightly beaten eggs
- 2 1/4 cups self-raising sifted flour (it is the flour with baking powder and salt added)

Direction:
1. Mix butter, milk, sugar, dates and spices in a pan, stir over heat until butter is melted, then bring to boil for a few seconds.
2. Remove from heat, stir in soda, set aside for about 5 minutes.
3. Stir in lightly beaten eggs and sifted flour in two lots. Then mix thoroughly.
4. Note: If you want to make your own self-rising flour, all you have to do is mix to 1 cup of all-purpose flour with 1 1/2 teaspoons of baking powder and 1/2 teaspoon of

salt. In our case, multiply everything by two.
5. Pour mixture into a greased 8-inch ring tin, bake on medium heat oven for 40 minutes.
6. Let it cool.

Joke:
- The best cure for coronavirus is having sex with a stranger in a white coat!
- Excuse me, are you a really therapist?

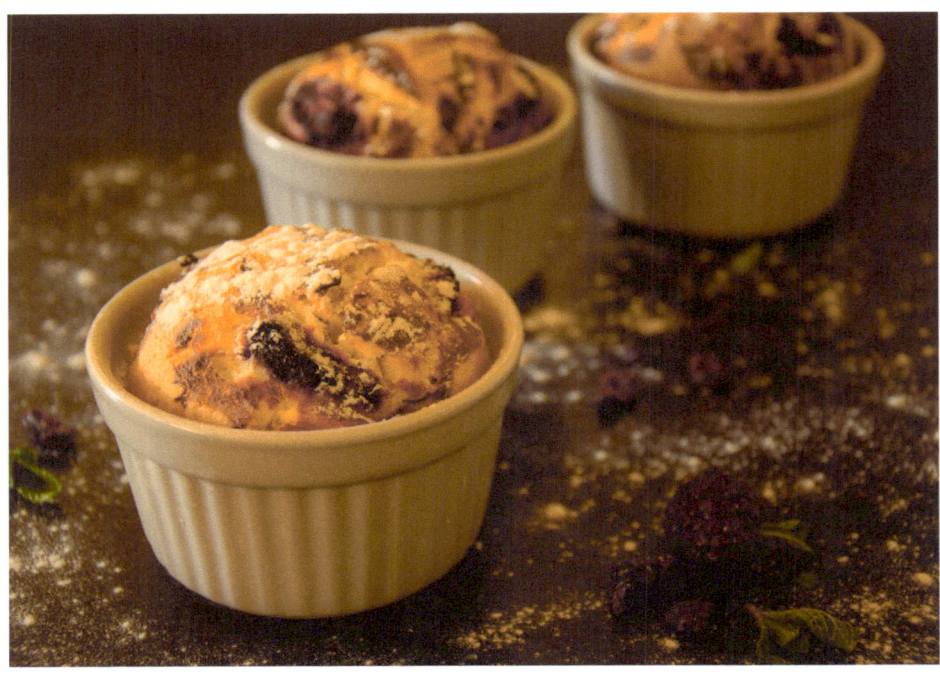

Have a good sex!

I recommend choosing one smoothie for yourself and drinking it for at least two weeks. So the body can get the most out of the components.

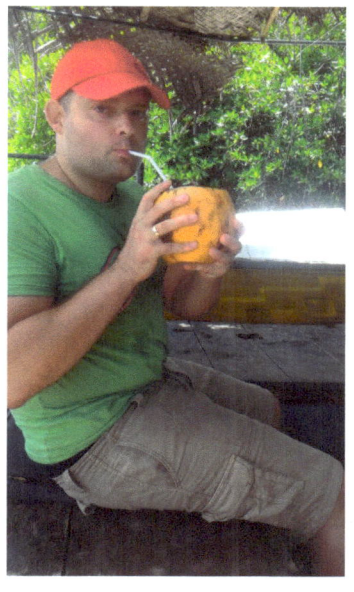

In addition, I recommend light physical exercise. If you do not have the time or desire to do gymnastics, you can just walk 30 minute per day. You can also take a prostate massage course.

For this, it is advisable to consult a specialist. This will help to clear the prostatic duct. It will significantly increase male potency and erection.

Goshua Iem

Goshua Iem

Text Copyright © 2020 Nestor Books

All rights reserved. No part of this book may be reproduced or transmitted in any form or by any means, electronic or mechanical, including photocopying, recording, or by an information storage and retrieval system - except by a reviewer who may quote brief passages in a review to be printed in a magazine or newspaper - without permission in writing from the publisher.

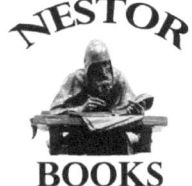

www.ingramcontent.com/pod-product-compliance
Lightning Source LLC
Chambersburg PA
CBHW041944240526
45473CB00033B/508